C000077452

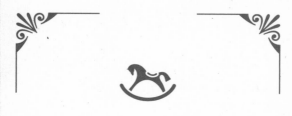

TOP TIPS

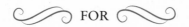

FOR

NEW GRANDPARENTS

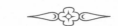

LOUISE BATY

summersdale

TOP TIPS FOR NEW GRANDPARENTS

Louise Baty has asserted her moral right to be identified as the author of this work in accordance with sections 77 and 78 of the Copyright, Designs and Patents Act 1988.

An Hachette UK Company
www.hachette.co.uk

Summersdale Publishers Ltd
Part of Octopus Publishing Group Limited
Carmelite House
50 Victoria Embankment
LONDON
EC4Y 0DZ
UK

www.summersdale.com

Printed and bound in the Czech Republic

ISBN: 978-1-78685-974-7

Substantial discounts on bulk quantities of Summersdale books are available to corporations, professional associations and other organizations. For details contact general enquiries: telephone: +44 (0) 1243 771107 or email: enquiries@summersdale.com.

Disclaimer
The information given in this book should not be treated as a substitute for qualified medical advice. Neither the author nor the publisher can be held responsible for any loss or claim arising out of the use, or misuse, of the suggestions made or the failure to take medical advice.

For Joan, Ros, Bill and
Morris – with love

CONTENTS

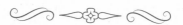

INTRODUCTION

Congratulations! You're going to be a new grandparent. Yes, really! It may not seem quite real yet and, as you embark on this wonderful stage in your life, you may feel a tad overwhelmed. After all, although you've been a parent, clearly this is uncharted territory.

Grandparenting is quite different from parenting (some actually consider it to be much more fun), so don't be alarmed if you are required to change your perspective, and approach, from the experiences of your own early parenting days.

With that in mind, it pays to be prepared before your grandchild makes an appearance and this book will help you do just that. From managing bath time and nappy changes to preparing bottle feeds and calming your new grandchild – along with everything in between – this book will outline the dos and don'ts of being a new grandparent.

It will also introduce you to new and interesting parenting trends, from baby showers to baby-led weaning. Divided into useful chapters, this book can be read and absorbed in one go or dipped into, as and when is needed. With your memory fully refreshed, you can get on with the important business of nurturing a close bond with your precious grandchild and thoroughly enjoying your important new role in life.

BEING SUPPORTIVE DURING THE PREGNANCY

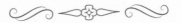

While pregnancy can be a magical time, it can also be fraught with worry. There's no doubt that parents-to-be need support from their families – both practical and emotional – in the run up to their baby's birth, even if they don't realize it initially.

OFFER EMOTIONAL SUPPORT

Never forget how anxiety-inducing pregnancy can be for parents-to-be. Morning sickness, fatigue, hospital appointment jitters and anxiety over the impending labour and birth...

It's a head spin, to say the least, so try to be as understanding and sympathetic as you can. First and foremost, be a parent. After all, you know your child like no one else – whether they're the one going through pregnancy or they're supporting their pregnant partner.

Follow your instincts when it comes to helping and supporting your child through this life-changing experience.

BE A SUPPORTIVE GRANDPARENT-TO-BE

Sometimes, parents-to-be can have difficult decisions to make during the pregnancy. In these circumstances, it's important not to interfere or judge. Just let them know you're there for them, no matter what, because the reassurance you can provide as a parent is second to none. Gauge the situation and be sensitive about how you can offer your help. For instance, a mum-to-be suffering health complications may need practical help beyond emotional support, and you may be able to assist by taking her to and from medical appointments.

Sometimes, expectant parents may simply need a shoulder to cry on and reassurance that "this too will pass". Some women suffer antenatal depression – an issue not as widely documented as postnatal depression, but equally traumatic. It can be hard for a mum-to-be to recognize that she's depressed, but if you see the signs – tearfulness, lack of energy, feeling isolated and chronically anxious – then do encourage them to seek professional help.

BE THERE WHEN
IT MATTERS

There's a chance you may be called upon to accompany the parents-to-be to medical appointments. You may be asked to help out with practical matters such as choosing cots or prams. If it's feasible, do your best to be there. Equally though, don't overstep the mark. Know when to stand back and take cues from the parents about when your help is really needed.

Be kind to yourself too. The truth is that seeing your child experiencing the highs and lows associated with pregnancy can be a testing time, so make sure to confide in a trusted relative or friend, if and when you feel the need.

SCANS – WHAT TO EXPECT

During ultrasound scans, there's usually only space in the scanning room for one extra adult aside from the sonographer and expectant mum. But if mum-to-be's partner can't attend, it's a good idea for her to have someone to support her – and that someone may be you!

Be aware that while scans can be exciting and reassuring, they can also be anxiety-inducing. Most UK mums-to-be have appointments at around weeks 12 and 20, but some may have earlier scans if they've experienced bleeding or previous miscarriages. Some may also opt for additional private scans.

Your role during the scan will be that of "emotional support", so be prepared to comfort mum-to-be if any issues arise. The fact is that while these appointments are a welcome chance to see that little bundle up on screen, some scans sadly reveal problems.

Ultrasound pregnancy scans are now standard, of course, but if you've never attended one, here are the basics:

◆ Scans are painless. Mum-to-be may feel pressure on her abdomen as the sonographer presses the handheld sensor on it.

◆ Mum-to-be will lie in a dimly lit room so the sonographer can see images on the screen.

◆ The sonographer may take 20 to 30 minutes to obtain all measurements and checks.

◆ Most hospitals provide a precious printout of the baby on the screen. Bring spare change to pay for it!

ANNOUNCEMENT
ETIQUETTE

There's only one rule for announcing the impending arrival: it's not your news to announce! See it from the point of view of the parents-to-be. This is their excitement. Their baby. Letting you in on their secret before telling their wider circle of family and friends doesn't mean you can spread the word before they've had the chance.

Many parents-to-be wait until after their 12-week scan before announcing the news – whether on social media or face to face. Some don't announce it publicly at all. Take your cues from them. Once they've told the wider world, then you can extend it to your circle too. When that moment comes, enjoy it… you're going to be a grandparent!

Sometimes our
grandmas and grandpas
are like grand-angels.

LEXIE SAIGE

PLANNING LABOUR – WHAT'S YOUR PLACE IN IT ALL?

You may be hovering anxiously by the phone once mum-to-be goes into labour, or you may be beside her in the delivery room. Either way, be prepared.

Waiting for news is agonizing, but resist the urge to keep calling for updates. It won't help anyone, least of all the stressed out parents-to-be.

If you've been asked to be a birthing partner, you'll be giving emotional support and reassurance during labour, as well as helping with breathing and relaxation techniques. Parents-to-be usually learn these techniques at antenatal classes. As a birthing partner, it may be useful for you to attend a class with mum-to-be, but if that's not possible, make sure she demonstrates them to you before the big day. It's also important to ask her to outline how she'd like you to help, before she goes into labour.

It's wise to have read her birth plan too, if she's written one. These days, parents-to-be are encouraged to outline the way they'd like their baby's birth to go. For example, they may envisage a water birth with minimal intervention. But in the event of labour not going as expected, medics caring for mum and baby will advise on the best course of action.

WHAT WILL YOU
BE CALLED?

Choosing your grandparenting name is one of life's small pleasures. It could also end up being an etiquette nightmare, especially if other grandparents are involved. What if both you and the other grandmother plump for "Granny"?

As always, speak to the new parents about it first, as they may have some ideas. You could invent your very own unique name or borrow from another language. For instance, Greek grandparents go by the fabulous "Yaya" and "Pappoús".

Bear in mind that, with all the best planning in the world, once your grandchild can talk, they may bestow on you their very own unique term of endearment. If that's the case, that'll be your name henceforth!

PLANNING A BABY SHOWER

Baby showers are becoming increasingly popular, but they're a relatively recent trend. You may well never have been invited to one, let alone organized one!

However, don't fret if the job of organizing a baby shower for mum-to-be has fallen to you.

Firstly, bear in mind that baby showers are something of an acquired taste. It's not everyone's cup of tea to be the centre of attention, especially when they're perilously close to their due date and can't see their feet. So it's always better to check first rather than throwing a surprise party. That said, baby showers can be the ideal opportunity for mum-to-be to spend time with loved ones before she disappears into a fog of nappies and sleepless nights…

Ideas for throwing the perfect baby shower:

◆ Choose a day well in advance of the due date to allow for an early arrival!

◆ When writing out invitations for the baby shower, consider specifying to guests that, if they wish to give a gift to the parents-to-be, more practical items would be appreciated, such as muslins or vouchers for baby supplies. Otherwise, they may end up with a mountain of soft toys.

◆ Ask guests to bring a copy of their favourite children's book. You'll be able to create a library for your grandchild that has lots of sentimental value.

◆ For decorations, how about bunting, balloons and baby photos of the parents-to-be?

◆ Shower the new family with love. Ask guests to write a wish for the baby's future, which you then put into a jar. Mum-to-be can read them during the party or take them home to enjoy.

◆ Try the "baby predictions" game, asking guests to guess the arrival date, gender (if this hasn't yet been found out) and weight of the baby.

Nobody can do for little children what grandparents do. Grandparents sort of sprinkle stardust over the lives of little children.

Alex Haley

WHEN TO GIVE YOUR OPINION AND WHEN TO STEP BACK

There are many decisions to make during pregnancy. Which cot? Which pram? Which name?

As the parents-to-be wade through a murky sea of indecision, it can be hard not to offer your own opinions.

But bear in mind that, for instance, baby name choices are more eclectic these days. While popular names in the 1980s included Michael and Jennifer, you're just as likely to meet a baby Rex or Pearl these days. A baby James might well be a girl, as gender neutral names are becoming popular.

Buggies are very different these days too – in fact, some parents eschew them altogether, preferring to carry their offspring in slings.

It's best to proceed with caution when it comes to offering your own guidance on parenting choices this early. Take cues from the parents about when your advice would be welcome.

The idea that no one
is perfect is a view
most commonly held
by people with no
grandchildren.

Doug Larson

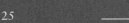

YOUR NOTES

....
....
....
....
....
....
....
....
....
....
....
....
....
....
....
....

YOUR NOTES

....
....
....
....
....
....
....
....
....
....
....
....
....
....
....
....

PREPARING FOR THE NEW ARRIVAL

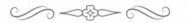

Hang out the bunting and get your home grandchild-ready! At some point in the not-so-distant future, your grandchild will be here. The chances are they'll be visiting you once the parents have found their feet a little. Knowing how to get your home grandchild-ready can be a confusing business, but this chapter will outline all the essentials.

MAKE A PLAN

Before your new grandchild's arrival, it's important to know how long and often they will stay with you, so you know exactly what you need. If baby will be visiting regularly and staying overnight, you might consider turning your spare room – if you have one – into a nursery. Alternatively, you could clear a space in your own bedroom or living room to accommodate your grandchild. For short visits, you will want to ensure you have the essentials. But, whatever your situation, don't feel you have to go overboard in purchasing a raft of new equipment – having the basics is enough.

However, there are some useful pieces of kit to consider, if baby's parents aren't providing their own during baby's stay. Make sure you consult with your grandchild's parents before you buy any "big ticket" item so that you know they're happy with your choice.

Here's a brief but certainly not exhaustive list of items you may need to buy:

◆ A Moses basket or cot. (See page 32.)

◆ A suitable car seat, if you're going to be driving your grandchild around. (See page 38.)

◆ An emergency stash of nappies, clothes, muslins, baby wipes, sterilized bottles and formula milk (if that's what baby has) is also handy.

◆ It's also wise to refresh your memory on changing bag "must haves". Clue: nappies, baby wipes and yet more nappies... See page 41 for more details.

Grandmas hold our tiny hands for just a little while, but our hearts forever.

Anonymous

WHERE WILL BABY SLEEP?

Newborns will happily doze in their pram or buggy or in someone's warm and cosy arms. But if they're staying overnight, you'll need something suitable for longer sleeps. Firstly, before buying anything discuss it with the parents-to-be to ensure that they're happy with the make and specifications.

Ensure your cot, crib or Moses basket conforms to British safety standards (BSEN716). Moses baskets and cribs are only suitable for the first few months until baby can pull themselves up. If you opt for a cot, experts recommend bars on all four sides so air can circulate. Bars should be vertical and no more than 6.5 cm (2.5 in) apart to prevent baby's head getting wedged. A foldable travel cot is a good option if you don't have space for a permanent cot.

Digging out an old family heirloom may seem like a lovely idea, but ensure it's safe to use. Some vintage cots may have been decorated with lead paint, for instance. Avoid old or second-hand mattresses which may contain nasties including mould, bacteria and dust mites. Some research has found a link between second-hand mattresses and SIDS (cot death). Ensure the mattress you choose feels firm, not soft, and conforms to safety standards.

Duvets and pillows are now considered suffocation hazards, along with cot bumpers and soft toys. Baby sleeping bags are seen as the safest option.

If you're transforming your spare room into a nursery, finish redecorating well before baby is due to visit. Little ones shouldn't sleep in a newly painted room in case they inhale fumes. Low VOC or VOC-free paints are best, as they contain less solvents than regular paints.

Maintain a room temperature of 16 to 20°C (68 to 72°F) to avoid your grandchild overheating. You may find a digital room thermometer and a baby monitor are useful purchases.

FUN IDEAS FOR A
VISITING GRANDCHILD

There's a wealth of items available to keep your new grandchild entertained, and it's tempting to try to provide them with everything you can. However, take time to think about additions that are both fun and practical for when your grandchild comes to visit. For instance, a sensory toy might be more welcome than a huge cuddly bear, or a soothing night light might be a more practical addition than a mobile that could be tricky to hang. Take time to think things through rather than making impulse purchases.

One of the most
powerful handclasps is
that of a new grandbaby
around the finger
of a grandfather.

Joy Hargrove

FIRST TOYS

Newborns don't need much entertainment. Once they've learnt to focus, they'll enjoy being cuddled and looking at various adoring faces. Fast forward a few weeks and they'll love musical toys and anything with high-contrast colours. From four to six months, they'll start to grasp objects. Rattles, wooden rings and soft toys with tags are ideal. Why not fill a small basket with a selection?

Bear in mind that babies put everything in their mouths, so clean toys regularly and be aware of choking hazards. Never let young children play with uninflated or broken balloons and avoid balls or other items smaller than 4.5 cm (1.75 in) in diameter.

CHOOSING THE RIGHT CAR SEAT

If you're likely to be driving your grandchild around on a regular basis, it might be worth buying a car seat for your vehicle. The world of baby car seats can be perplexing so it's important to do your research.

◆ Never buy a second-hand car seat. There's no way of knowing whether it's been involved in an accident, making it unsafe.

◆ Understand how the sizing categories work – you'll see group numbers alongside each model of car seat you browse. These groups accommodate a particular age range and weight. When shopping for a newborn car seat in the UK, the only group numbers to concern yourself with are Group 0, which lasts approximately from birth to six to nine months (0–10 kg/0–22 lbs) and Group 0+, which lasts approximately from birth to 12 to 15 months (0–13 kg/0–29 lbs).

◆ All babies must be in a rear-facing seat until they're 15 months old. Before this age, their necks aren't strong enough to withstand a head-on collision in a forward-facing seat.

◆ Some car seats can be secured with the seat belt. However, the ISOFIX system – the international standard for attachment points for child safety seats in passenger cars – is seen as a safer method of installation. Car seats are clicked firmly into place at fixed anchor points. The system is known as LATCH in the USA and LUAS in Canada. Be warned that not all ISOFIX car seats fit all ISOFIX-enabled cars. So do your homework and check that your chosen seat is compatible with your vehicle.

A child needs a grandparent, anybody's grandparent, to grow a little more securely into an unfamiliar world.

CHARLES AND ANN MORSE

BEING PREPARED WHEN YOU'RE OUT AND ABOUT

When you're out and about with your son/daughter and grandchild, they will most likely have a fully-prepared baby bag ready for any eventuality. But let's face it, sleep deprivation causes forgetfulness and new parents are bound to wander out of the house in a fog of confusion, without a ready supply of nappies, at some point or other. It might be useful for you to save the day by carrying emergency wipes or spare nappies just in case.

If you're in charge of packing the changing bag before a trip out, here's a useful, although by no means exhaustive, list:

- Bottles and milk, if required

- Muslins

- Foldable changing mat

- Nappies

- Wet wipes (environmentally friendly biodegradable or reusable versions are available)

- Nappy cream

- Nappy bags

- Hand sanitizer

- At least one spare outfit for baby

- A spare top for yourself, if you'd rather not model patches of baby sick on your clothes in public!

BABYPROOFING YOUR HOME

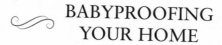

Newborns can't get up to much mischief by themselves, but the best time for babyproofing your home is well before your grandchild's due date, so you can give it proper thought. Initial precautions are to ensure adults in charge of baby stay safe. Heaven forbid anyone slips or trips when carrying that precious bundle! So fit non-slip mats under all rugs and move trailing wires from electrical objects well away from where anyone will tread.

Install carbon monoxide and smoke alarms, purchase a fire extinguisher (and know how to use it) and fit a temperature guard on your water heater to prevent scalding accidents. Stock up your first aid supplies too.

By law, all plug sockets must be wired in with safety shutters to prevent tiny fingers accessing live terminals, so socket covers aren't necessary, but this is, of course, at your discretion.

Once baby is crawling (from around six months), you'll need a second "risk assessment". This is the time to fit baby gates on stairs, check window locks, remove blinds with looped cords and remove or secure tall wobbly furniture, such as lamps or chests of drawers.

You should also cover sharp furniture edges with guards and move anything potentially dangerous – knives, scissors, medicines and cleaning fluids – out of reach. It's also time to cast an eye over all areas that baby might roam to make sure tiny objects are removed, as they like to explore and discover their world by putting things in their mouth. Be extra vigilant to remove any choking hazards.

YOUR NOTES

....
....
....
....
....
....
....
....
....
....
....
....
....
....
....
....
....

YOUR NOTES

....
....
....
....
....
....
....
....
....
....
....
....
....
....

OFFERING EMOTIONAL SUPPORT

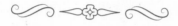

Your grandchild has finally
arrived – it's time to celebrate!
But do spare a thought for the
new parents who may well be
feeling overwhelmed and in need
of your support and guidance.

Grandchildren are God's
way of compensating
us for growing old.

Mary H. Waldrip

STRAIGHT AFTER THE BIRTH – WHAT TO EXPECT

Once baby has safely arrived, everyone can breathe a sigh of relief, right? Yes, of course – but it's important to recognize that the rigours of labour and birth – especially the first time – can leave new parents feeling a little shell-shocked in the early days.

Even if you have, yourself, given birth in the past, recognize that every single woman's experience is different. Along with the welfare of your precious grandchild in the early days, mum's recovery and well-being is paramount.

Around 80 per cent of new mums experience the baby blues in some form, which leave them feeling weepy, emotional and irritable. Then there's the worry of a whole new responsibility, which can also hit hard. And don't forget mum's partner in all this.

The arrival of your precious grandchild is to be celebrated, of course. But be understanding if the new parents seem a tad overwhelmed.

PLANNING YOUR FIRST VISIT

Once baby's arrived, hang on until you zoom over to the hospital or family home, if baby was a home birth. Mum and baby will be recovering, for starters, and may be having further treatment.

Check the hospital's rules on visitors but, most importantly, check what the new parents want. If it's okay for you to visit, make sure you know what you're allowed to take. Most hospitals don't allow flowers due to risk of infections.

If you're meeting baby at home, bear in mind that some new parents prefer a few quiet days before the wider family descends. Respect their wishes and wait until they're ready for you to enjoy those newborn cuddles.

HELPING NEW
PARENTS COPE WITH
BROKEN NIGHTS

Babies are super cute, but they have a tendency to spring awake at 3 a.m. and they certainly don't respect lie-ins! Sleep deprivation, after having a baby, can be earth shattering. There you are, enjoying eight hours' sleep each night when… boom! You're suddenly being woken at two-hourly intervals. Not fun.

But of course, it's totally normal, so reassure the new parents that this stage is all par for the course and will eventually pass. If possible, offer hands-on assistance. Turning up in the wee hours probably isn't workable. Why not offer to babysit during the day instead? That way, the new parents can slope off for a much needed nap.

If I had known how
wonderful it would be
to have grandchildren,
I'd have had them first.

Lois Wyse

GUIDING NEW PARENTS
THROUGH THEIR WORRIES

Realizing it's your job to look after a newborn 24/7 can be overwhelming. But new parents often put on a brave face, for fear of people thinking they "can't cope". Explain that parenting is not about perfection; it's about learning "on the job". Offer your advice and guidance, but reiterate that they're already doing fantastically.

Sometimes, anxieties run deeper than the usual baby blues. Postnatal depression and postnatal anxiety affect up to one in every ten new mums in the first year. If you suspect your grandchild's mum – or dad – may be suffering, reassure them that help is available and encourage them to speak to a health professional.

HELPING
NEW PARENTS
❦ COPE WITH ❦
RELATIONSHIP
CHANGES

Becoming parents is one of the biggest life changes a couple can face. Many couples struggle with having less "quality time" together. It's hard to get romantic with a tiny person between you – sometimes literally!

Lack of sleep can lead to frayed tempers and "exhaustion one-upmanship", e.g. "You can't possibly be more tired than me…"

Some new parents – male and female – struggle to adjust to the new reality that their baby is their main focus. And, if one parent is taking a career break to look after baby full time, there may be concerns over finances. As always, be understanding and kind.

Many couples find it hard to confide in their loved ones when it comes to relationship issues. It can be too personal – too raw – to share, so it's important not to interfere. But if you notice that the new parents may be struggling, it might help to offer the wisdom of your own experience. Reassure them that this time will pass – that "couple time" will return at some point.

If you can offer practical help, do. Even the odd hour of babysitting is worth its weight in gold. It means the new parents can head to the local café for a quick lunch and catch-up.

If the relationship is in danger of breaking down, it may be useful to suggest relationship counselling, depending on circumstance.

Grandparents are
a delightful blend
of laughter, caring
deeds, wonderful
stories and love.

Anonymous

YOUR NOTES

....
....
....
....
....
....
....
....
....
....
....
....
....
....
....
....

YOUR NOTES

....
....
....
....
....
....
....
....
....
....
....
....
....
....
....
....

OFFERING PRACTICAL SUPPORT

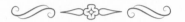

Whether you can batch cook meals for the new parents, offer financial support, do some tidying or cleaning or just hold the baby for a while to give them a break, your hands-on help will be appreciated.

Grandma always made you feel she had been waiting to see just you all day and now the day was complete.

MARCY DEMAREE

HOW TO BE A
USEFUL VISITOR

New parents can feel inundated with visitors who monopolize their sofa, drinking tea, eating biscuits and cuddling the baby – leaving a mess of empty mugs and dirty plates in their wake.

Don't be that visitor! As tempting as it is to sit for hours, holding the baby, try to make yourself useful. You could:

- have a quick tidy, chucking out obvious rubbish (always check first!)
- do the washing-up or load the dishwasher
- empty the bins and take out the recycling
- clean the bathroom
- stick a load of washing in the machine
- do some ironing.

What a bargain
grandchildren are!
I give them my loose
change, and they give
me a million dollars'
worth of pleasure.

GENE PERRET

GIVE THEM SOME "ME TIME"

Most new parents find themselves unable to do the sorts of mundane things they once took for granted, so sometimes holding the baby is actually JUST the right thing to do.

With a little one permanently clamped to you, you find yourselves aching to nip to the toilet, make a quick cup of tea, flop on the sofa or have an uninterrupted bath or shower! So go over there, take baby into another room or for a walk in their buggy and let their parent reclaim a bit of "me time", even if it's only for an hour or two. It will make their day.

COOK UP A STORM

When it comes to the tasks occupying a new parent's mind, feeding themselves often comes way down the list. In fact, many new mums and dads find themselves existing on cups of cold tea and microwave meals. But new parents – especially breastfeeding mums – need regular, nutritious, filling meals.

Why not make them a home-cooked meal which can be heated in the oven? Lasagne, chilli and cottage pie are great ideas. Homemade soup which can be heated up in a pan is also a winner. Or batch cook meals such as stew or curry, which can be frozen in individual portions and then defrosted and heated, as required. Vouchers for grocery deliveries or takeaways might also be appreciated.

OFFER FINANCIAL HELP

Finances can be tight for new parents. If you're financially able, why not contribute toward one of the "big ticket" items during pregnancy, such as the pram or cot? Alternatively, buy a bundle of useful "must haves" such as multipacks of wet wipes and nappies.

The parents may also have the cost of childcare to consider, which can be astronomical. If you're able to care for your grandchild on a regular or ad hoc basis, rest assured you'd be saving them a huge amount.

Of course, for many grandparents-to-be, it's just not feasible to contribute financially. Rest assured that your practical and emotional support will mean more to your grandchild's parent than any monetary gifts.

OFFER A LEGACY GIFT

The excitement of a new grandchild can make it tempting to shower the newborn with gifts. However, if you know that space is a premium at home why not consider a legacy gift, something that your grandchild will grow up to cherish and remember you by? There are so many different ideas to choose from. For example, you could open up a bank account for a newborn, where you contribute small amounts for special occasions – they'll thank you for the cash in the long term. Or maybe you would like to offer your grandchild the gift of altruism by supporting a charity in some way.

There are countless causes that can be supported, from sponsoring a child or an animal in need, to planting a tree that will help the environment and grow with them. Whatever you decide upon, you can provide information about the gift that your grandchild can read in due course when they are able to comprehend the true value of your offering.

If nothing is going well,
call your grandmother.

ITALIAN PROVERB

MAKE A MEMORY

When a new baby arrives in a family, the cameras invariably appear too. Everyone wants a pic of themselves with the precious bundle, but don't forget the parents. After all, this is one of the most memorable times of their lives. Snap some family shots of them together, then send the photos to them. Even better, print them out, old school style, so they don't have to bother doing it themselves.

If you have a tendency to take out-of-focus pics, why not pay for a professional photo shoot of the family? It's a gift they'd treasure.

On the subject of photos, remember it's considered polite to ask parents for permission before you post photos of their children on social media.

Other ways to make memories:

◆ Write a letter to your grandchild, telling them about themselves as a newborn and the special people in their lives. Some new parents make memory boxes for their children, filled with keepsakes to look at when they're older. A letter from you would be a wonderful addition.

◆ Write a card or letter to the new parents telling them how well they're doing in their new role and how proud you are of them. It'll mean the world to them.

◆ Suggest making baby foot and hand prints. You can buy DIY kits or have them professionally done – a very thoughtful gift.

When a child is born,
so are grandmothers.

JUDITH LEVY

YOUR NOTES

....
....
....
....
....
....
....
....
....
....
....
....
....
....
....

YOUR NOTES

....
....
....
....
....
....
....
....
....
....
....
....
....
....

CARING FOR YOUR NEW GRANDCHILD

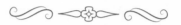

Quality hands-on time with your gorgeous grandchild is precious, but can be daunting at first. It's a huge responsibility, after all, and it's probably been a while since you last had to be so hands-on. The following notes will help you brush up on the basics of feeding, nappy changing and washing.

FEEDING TIME

We discuss feeding the baby in more detail in the next chapter, but here are some starter points:

◆ You'll recall that young babies feed regularly – every two hours or so, in the very early days – so you need to be prepared.

◆ If possible, the parents should provide written instructions which you can refer to once you're temporarily in charge.

◆ If your grandchild is breastfed, the parents will need to give you supplies of expressed milk. For pointers on preparing expressed milk feeds, go to page 99.

◆ If your grandchild is formula-fed, the parents should provide you with ample supplies and instructions. For further information on this, see page 100.

HOW TO BOTTLE FEED

Hold your grandchild fairly upright, making sure their head is supported. Brush the bottle teat against their lips until they open their mouth. Feeds can take a while so enjoy holding your grandchild and sharing this special time. For more guidance, look at Chapter Six – Feeding your new grandchild (page 94).

HOW TO CHANGE A NAPPY

Young babies need changing up to 10 to 12 times daily so it's good to know the basics.

◆ Be prepared with a changing mat or towel, cotton wool and warm water, or baby wipes, a plastic bag or bin, barrier cream and a clean nappy.

◆ Lay baby on the changing mat or towel. If you're using a changing table, don't leave them unattended.

◆ Wash your hands. Then remove the dirty nappy and use wipes or cotton wool and warm water to clean baby's bottom. Remember to clean inside folds of skin.

- Always clean baby girls from front to back to avoid infections. Clean around baby boys' genitals but don't pull back the foreskin.

- Use barrier cream and, if you have time, leave baby nappy free for a little while – this reduces the chance of nappy rash.

- Soiled disposable nappies can be rolled up and resealed using the tabs.

- Washable cloth nappies don't have to be soaked before washing but it may help remove stains. Always check washing instructions.

There's no place like
home except Grandma's.

ANONYMOUS

TOPPING AND TAILING

Babies don't need to be bathed every day, but if your grandchild needs a bit of a clean up when they are in your care here's a reminder about "topping and tailing".

Here's how:

◆ Fill a bowl with warm water and have cotton wool to hand.

◆ Lay baby on a warm towel on a changing mat or on your knee.

◆ Remove their clothes, except for their nappy and vest.

◆ Dip a piece of cotton wool in the water but don't get it sodden. Wipe gently around baby's eyes, from the nose outward. Use a clean piece of cotton wool on each eye.

◆ Clean around baby's ears, using clean cotton wool each time. Never wash inside or use cotton buds inside baby's ears.

◆ Gently wash the rest of baby's face, neck and hands and pat them dry gently with the towel.

◆ Remove baby's nappy and gently clean their bottom with damp cotton pads.

◆ Pat baby dry with a soft towel. Don't forget to dry between skinfolds and creases before putting on a clean nappy and clothes.

Love is the greatest gift
that one generation
can leave to another.

RICHARD GARNETT

BATH TIME

Bath time can be magical for you and for your little water baby, but make sure you're well prepared. Plastic baby baths are bulky to store so you may prefer a plastic or sponge bath support to place inside your own bath. With baby lying safely in the support, your hands are free to wash them. Of course, many people manage perfectly well washing their baby in the kitchen or bathroom sink! Back in your day, this may well have been standard, but it's a good idea to check with baby's parents first.

Also make sure you're confident in your ability to handle such precious, slippery cargo. When in doubt, err on the side of caution. It's best not to bathe baby straight after a feed or when they're tired or hungry.

Make sure the room is warm and that you have a towel to hand as well as a fresh nappy and clean clothes. The bath water should be warm but not hot – test it with your elbow and mix it to eradicate hot spots. It's best not to use products on babies under a month old. You can simply wash their skin and hair in clean water. If they're older, use bath products formulated for babies.

Never ever leave baby unattended in the bath, even momentarily.

Surely, two of the most
satisfying experiences
in life must be those
of being a grandchild
or a grandparent.

Donald A. Norberg

MAKE BEDTIME A SUCCESS

It may be tempting to keep baby up as long as possible so that you can have more of those lovely cuddles. But, as you probably know, overtired, overstimulated babies are a recipe for a disaster and will struggle to get to sleep – and stay asleep too.

So it's important to stick to your grandchild's nap and bedtime routine. As always, check with the parents so that you know how this routine pans out. But generally, it will go something along these lines:

- Bath time

- Change baby into bedtime clothes

- Bedtime milk feed

- Brush their teeth – if they have any, that is! (Some babies get their first teeth at four months although most don't see teeth appearing until six months. If their first teeth haven't appeared, you can brush their gums with a soft cloth or gauze after each feed but always check with the parents first.)

- Read them a story

- Listen to lullabies

- Enjoy a cuddle before bed

DON'T OVERSTEP THE LINE

When you're temporarily "in charge" of your grandchild, never forget that you're NOT the parent. Don't make big decisions without first consulting with your grandchild's parents – and, most importantly, respecting their views.

As obvious as it may sound, there are certain things it's inappropriate for anyone but the parents to make the decision to do. These include:

◆ Taking baby for their first haircut

◆ Piercing baby's ears

◆ Giving baby their very first foods if they haven't yet been weaned

◆ Trying baby on new foods, if they're being weaned

◆ Giving baby a dummy if they've previously never had one

89

POINTERS FOR SAFE SLEEPING

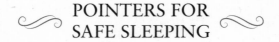

For the first six months, it's advisable for baby to sleep in a cot in the same room as you, but not in the same bed. Experts advise that babies are not put to sleep on their fronts, as tummy sleeping is thought to increase the risk of Sudden Infant Death Syndrome (SIDS).

Always place baby on their back, with their feet at the bottom of the cot, so they can't wriggle underneath bedding. Well-fitting baby sleeping bags are considered the safest way to keep baby warm at night, rather than loose blankets. The room temperature should be between 16 and 20°C (68 and 72°F).

If you're in charge overnight, brace yourself for a few wake ups. But remember that it's normal for babies to wake up at intervals during the night. If they've woken crying, check whether it's because they need a nappy change or milk feed. Sometimes, simply a cuddle or reassuring patting on their back will settle them enough for them to drift back to sleep.

Never leave baby's bottle in the cot with them, and allowing babies to suck on a bottle while going to sleep can increase the chance of "bottle rot" – tooth decay – as the teeth are being "bathed" in milk overnight.

YOUR NOTES

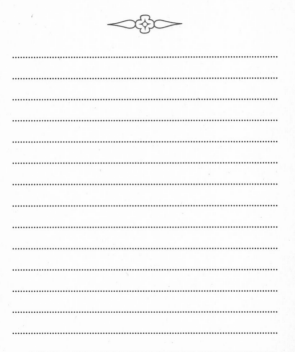

....
....
....
....
....
....
....
....
....
....
....
....
....
....
....
....

YOUR NOTES

....
....
....
....
....
....
....
....
....
....
....
....
....
....
....
....

FEEDING YOUR
NEW GRANDCHILD

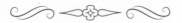

Breastfeeding or formula? Baby-led weaning or spooning mushy puree into that adorable little mouth? Choices, choices… However your grandchild's parents are opting to feed their little one, it's wise for you to be au fait with the basics.

I loved their home.
Everything smelled
older, worn but safe; the
food aroma had baked
itself into the furniture.

SUSAN STRASBERG ON
HER GRANDPARENTS

DO YOUR RESEARCH

There are fewer more divisive topics than the debate over breast versus bottle. As a grandparent, it's probably safer to stay well out of any such discussions. Accept that, however your grandchild's parents opt to feed their newborn, your role – as with most things grandparental – should be supportive, not judgemental.

That said, if you're asked for your advice, it's good to do your research on the basics, as well as knowing how to tackle potential feeding hurdles such as wind, reflux and tongue-tie.

And while experts recommend that babies aren't introduced to solid foods until around six months – which may seem a long way off if your grandchild hasn't even arrived yet – it's wise to start planning for this momentous step well in advance too.

Grandparents make
the world a little
softer, a little kinder
and a little warmer.

Anonymous

BREASTFEEDING –
HOW TO BE SUPPORTIVE

You'll maybe remember that newborns feed frequently and for up to 45 minutes at a time, which will take up a lot of mum's day. Some newborns latch on and never look back, but breastfeeding isn't simple for everyone. It can take weeks – months, even – to get into a rhythm. There's nothing worse than an audience when mum's settling her little one for a feed, so be supportive but never overbearing.

Breastfeeding mums use up to 700 calories a day producing breast milk. This means that they should consume 400 to 500 extra calories a day – preferably nutritious snacks such as chunks of cheese with carrot sticks, apple slices covered in peanut butter or raspberries with some pieces of good quality dark chocolate. So do bring some when you visit!

Breastfeeding will also leave mum thirsty, but it can be hard for her to find time to make drinks when she's focused on her little one. So if you find yourself at a loose end during feed times, focus on keeping mum's drink permanently topped up. This will prevent her becoming dehydrated, which can lead to constipation and urine infections.

Many mums express and freeze their breast milk so their babies can be bottle fed by others. If you're preparing frozen expressed milk, thaw it by placing the container in warm water and use it within 24 hours. If you want to warm the milk, place the container in warm water. Never warm it in the microwave as this can cause hot spots. Test the milk on the inside of your wrist before giving it to baby – it should be room temperature.

If God had intended us
to follow recipes, He
wouldn't have given
us grandmothers.

LINDA HENLEY

FORMULA FEEDING –
HOW TO PREPARE BOTTLES

When it comes to preparing formula feeds, there is a basic process to follow, although you must check the manufacturer's instructions and always use your grandchild's regular brand of formula, as approved by their parents. Here are some must dos and don'ts when it comes to preparing formula feeds.

◆ Wash your hands and sterilize surfaces, bottles and teats.

◆ Boil some water, using fresh tap water only. Bottled water isn't recommended for making up formula feeds as it's not sterile.

◆ After boiling the water, leave it to cool in the kettle for no more than half an hour, so that it remains at least 70°C (160°F). Water at this temperature kills any harmful bacteria.

◆ Only ever use the correct scoop for the brand of formula to avoid measuring mistakes. Don't add extra formula powder to the water as it may cause your grandchild to suffer constipation or dehydration.

◆ Test the temperature of the milk on the inside of your wrist before giving it to baby. It should be body temperature.

◆ To reduce the risk of infections from bacteria, it's best to make up feeds as needed rather than storing them up.

◆ Never add solid foods, such as baby rice, to baby's bottle feed as it's a choking hazard.

Grandparents,
like heroes, are as
necessary to a child's
growth as vitamins.

Joyce Allston

TACKLING FEEDING PROBLEMS

Remember that some babies experience early feeding difficulties, so it's best to be clued up just in case:

◆ Tongue-tie – known medically as ankyloglossia, tongue-tie affects 4 to 11 per cent of newborns and is more common in boys. Some babies with tongue-tie struggle to breastfeed because they can't latch on properly. Mums with tongue-tied babies may suffer sore nipples, mastitis or engorgement. Tongue-tie can be treated with a frenotomy, during which the frenulum is cut. It's quick and recovery is usually speedy.

◆ Reflux – bringing up milk during or after feeds is known as posseting or reflux. It isn't usually reason for concern, but it can cause babies to gag, refuse feeds, suffer persistent coughs, hiccups or ear infections and may also hinder weight gain. It can also indicate more serious issues such as allergies, so it's wise for baby's parents to consult a doctor if they have concerns.

◆ Wind and colic – these common issues are discussed in greater length on the next pages.

TACKLING WIND

Many babies may be plagued by painful wind which can make them very upset after having their milk. Wind is caused by air bubbles in baby's tummy, which they can't release by themselves. Two ways to wind your grandchild are:

- to put them over your shoulder and rub their back until they bring up air, or

- to sit them on your lap, facing away from you, while you straighten their back and rub it.

The parents should be able to tell you how best to wind your grandchild. Otherwise you'll hopefully work out which approach they prefer.

UNDERSTANDING COLIC

Some experts think colic pain is caused by air stretching the stomach. If you're not sure whether colic pain is bothering your grandchild, know the signs.

Is your grandchild:

◆ crying persistently and/or for long stretches of time, often starting in the early evening?

◆ clenching their fists?

◆ arching their back?

◆ drawing their knees up to their tummy?

If so, they might be suffering colic pain.

Over-the-counter colic relief medications are available. Other ideas for soothing a colicky baby include rocking them in your arms, taking them for a walk in their buggy, massaging them and playing soothing "white noise" (which we'll explain further in Chapter Seven on page 122). Thankfully, most babies overcome colic by around six months. Until then, when you're caring for your colicky grandchild, you may find it stressful. If you can, arrange for someone else to be there with you while you're caring for your grandchild so that they can take over comforting duties for a few minutes to give you a break.

INTRODUCING SOLIDS

Experts recommend that babies aren't introduced to solid foods before six months, but most parents start planning for the transition beforehand. It's important to be clued up on it all, as things may have changed.

Spoon feeding is still the most common technique today, with parents offering freshly pureed "first foods" or purees from jars. But baby-led weaning (BLW) is also gaining ground. This method allows babies to feed themselves right from the beginning. Although it may sound confusing, you simply have to offer baby a selection of age-appropriate finger foods, such as cooked spears of broccoli, slices of avocado and slices of banana (cut lengthways). They're easy for baby to grasp with their fists, lift to their mouths and suck.

Whether you're BLW or spoon feeding, it's vital to know about choking hazards. Babies can choke on foods including sausages, nuts, pieces of meat, boiled sweets, popcorn, raw vegetables, chunks of peanut butter, slices of apple and whole grapes so avoid these. Foods you give your grandchild to start with should be soft enough for them to squash between finger and thumb.

For steps on dealing with a choking baby, there's a tip at the end of this chapter. Also, remember that experts advise against giving sugar to babies under a year old. As always, check with the parents first before trying any new food on your grandchild.

WHAT TO DO IF BABY IS CHOKING

Always watch your grandchild when they're eating and know the difference between gagging and choking. Gagging is noisy whereas choking is, more often than not, silent. Here's a step-by-step guide to what to do if your grandchild is choking.

◆ First lay baby face down on your thigh, supporting their head. Using the heel of your hand, hit them firmly on the back between their shoulder blades. Repeat up to five times.

◆ Turn baby over, lying them face up on your thigh. Look in their mouth and pick out any obvious objects.

◆ If baby is still choking, keep them lying face up on your thigh. Place two fingers in the middle of their chest and push sharply downward. Repeat up to five times.

◆ If the obstruction still hasn't cleared, call for emergency help. While waiting for help, keep trying to clear the obstruction using back blows followed by chest thrusts.

Grandchildren are the
dots that connect the
lines from generation
to generation.

Lois Wyse

YOUR NOTES

....
....
....
....
....
....
....
....
....
....
....
....
....
....
....

YOUR NOTES

....
....
....
....
....
....
....
....
....
....
....
....
....
....
....
....

CALMING YOUR NEW GRANDCHILD

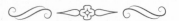

No matter how well prepared
you are, all sensible thoughts may
fly out of the window once your
grandchild's in your arms and
they won't stop crying. Brush up
on tried and tested methods for
soothing that precious bundle,
without stressing yourself out too.

Grandchildren give
us a second chance
to do things better
because they bring
out the best in us.

Anonymous

REMEMBER THAT CRYING IS NORMAL

◆ As you may recall, newborns cry up to two to three hours a day – and this is completely normal. Some babies may seem more "fussy" than others and the truth is that some are more sensitive to new noises, smells or people.

◆ Newborns' cries sound very high-pitched and "frantic" because they're taking in short breaths between cries. Their cries will become longer and louder as they get older.

◆ When you're faced with your seemingly inconsolable grandchild, try not to panic that you're doing anything wrong – or that it's somehow your fault. It's not!

◆ Be aware that "cry it out" – a method of "sleep training" in which babies are left to cry themselves to sleep – is highly controversial. Most experts agree that babies need comfort and reassurance when in distress.

CHECK THE BASICS

When your grandchild's crying, don't leap to conclusions and panic that there's something dreadfully wrong. First things first, check the basics.

◆ HUNGRY? If they're squirming and their cries are getting increasingly loud, that could be the answer.

◆ DIRTY NAPPY? If you can't smell the evidence, have a quick look. Newborns need their nappies changed up to 10 to 12 times a day.

◆ WIND? Piercing wails can mean they're in pain, possibly from wind.

◆ TOO HOT OR TOO COLD? The room where baby is sleeping should be between 16 and 20°C (68 and 72°F). A digital room thermometer may be useful.

Grandparents are similar to a piece of string – handy to have around and easily wrapped around the fingers of their grandchildren.

Anonymous

TACKLING COLIC AND WIND

As we've already discussed in the previous chapter, these common problems can cause real distress to babies.

Wind is thought to be caused by air bubbles forming in babies' stomachs, which they're unable to expel by themselves. Some experts say that colic is caused by air stretching babies' stomachs. It's good to remember that most babies overcome colic by around six months. Until then, when you're caring for your colicky grandchild, you may find it stressful. If you can, arrange for someone else to be there with you while you're on babysitting duties so that they can take over comforting duties for a few minutes to give you a break.

For tips on tackling wind and colic, read the tips on pages 106 and 107.

THE POWER OF WHITE NOISE

Similar to radio static, white noise helps to send babies to sleep. It's soothing, quite simply, because it reminds them of being tucked safely in the womb, when sounds were muffled by amniotic fluid.

Just as you may repeatedly whisper "ssshh" to settle your grandchild, playing white noise can reassure and soothe them. In fact, researchers found that it helped 80 per cent of babies fall asleep within five minutes!

If you don't have a radio to hand, you can download white noise apps on your phone. Other constant background noise such as a vacuum cleaner may have the same soothing effect.

CALMING WITH MOTION

Babies are soothed by motion because it reminds them of being in the womb. Try these methods:

◆ Rock them in your arms. Standing up is usually easiest. Sway side to side with them and watch them relax.

◆ Take them for a walk in their buggy. The motion should soon send them off to sleep.

◆ Try a sling. Stretchy wraps tend to suit newborns, while structured carriers work better for older babies. Slings leave your hands free while baby snuggles into your chest. Check with your grandchild's parents, use a reputable brand and read the instructions properly before using the equipment.

◆ Go for a drive. Car seats and babies are a recipe for naps.

◆ Put baby in a rocking baby chair or crib.

HOW TO SWADDLE A BABY

Swaddling has been used for centuries in some cultures and is becoming increasingly widespread. It's thought to lessen the effect of the baby's startle reflex and remind them of feeling secure in the womb. But experts warn that if you're going to swaddle a baby, you must start at birth and do it consistently. So never try swaddling your grandchild without having first checked with the parents that it's something they're already doing.

Other pointers are:

◆ Always use a thin sheet.

◆ Leave baby's head uncovered and don't swaddle above the shoulders.

◆ Never place baby on their side or front. They must be on their back.

◆ Don't swaddle if baby is showing signs of rolling onto their tummy.

◆ Swaddle firmly but not tightly so that baby's legs and feet can move freely and bend at the hip.

◆ Check baby's temperature regularly as overheating can increase the risk of SIDS (cot death).

Truth be told, being a grandma is as close as we ever get to perfection. The ultimate warm sticky bun with plump raisins and nuts. Clouds nine, ten, and eleven.

Bryna Nelson Paston

SING A LULLABY

You can't get more traditional than a lullaby. Don't worry – newborns won't notice if you can't hit the high notes. The old songs are the best – "Twinkle Twinkle Little Star" and "Rock-a-Bye Baby" have been calming babies for many years and still work just as well today. Hold your grandchild close and sing to them softly. It may help if you stand up and sway as you sing. Or you could sit in a cosy rocking chair and snuggle up.

Your little one is sure to calm down in no time and when they do, let time stand still and treasure the moment. If you'd rather not sing yourself, lullaby CDs are available to buy.

COPING WITH
SEPARATION ANXIETY

Don't take it personally if your grandchild wails when their parents leave you temporarily in charge. It's a normal stage of a child's development, as they become aware of the wider world.

Tackle separation anxiety by "starting small". Suggest looking after your grandchild for ten minutes at first, gradually building up the length of time that you're in sole charge. Baby may feel soothed by cuddling something they associate with their parents, such as a blanket or snuggle toy with their scent on it.

When it's time for baby's parents to leave, they should be positive and reassuring. By giving big smiles and promises to be "back soon", they'll help ease baby's fears.

WHEN TO SEEK MEDICAL HELP

Sometimes, baby is crying because they're ill and need medical attention. The best course of action is to notify the parents immediately so that they can decide how baby should be cared for. If the parents cannot care for the baby, book an appointment with a GP as soon as possible or seek an appointment with the out-of-hours doctor if your grandchild:

◆ is under three months and has a temperature over 38°C (100°F)

◆ is between three months and six months and has a temperature over 39°C (102°F)

◆ has had diarrhoea six times or more in the past 24 hours or diarrhoea lasting more than two days

129

◆ is vomiting repeatedly and bringing up green vomit or vomit streaked with blood

◆ is dehydrated (signs are dry lips and mouth, dark yellow urine, fewer wet nappies and sunken fontanelles (the soft spot on the top of baby's head))

◆ is under 28 days and has sticky, red eyes, which could be neonatal conjunctivitis

◆ has bleeding from their umbilical cord stump.

Seek immediate emergency care (by going to A&E or calling for an ambulance) if your grandchild:

◆ has a fever, despite having had baby paracetamol or ibuprofen, and is floppy and/ or drowsy

◆ has swallowed something harmful, such as adult medication or a lithium battery

- has a foreign object lodged in their ear or nose

- is having trouble breathing

- won't wake up or can't stay awake

- has a cut that may need stitching (stem the bleeding by pressing a clean cloth on the wound, until you get help)

- has a febrile convulsion (fit) caused by a fever

- has suffered a burn or scald

- is showing one or more signs of meningitis or septicaemia (fever with cold hands and feet, drowsiness, floppiness, crying or moaning, rapid breathing, grunting, swollen fontanelles, aversion to bright lights, pale blotchy skin or a purple-red rash that remains when you press a glass against it)

- is showing signs of sepsis (breathing difficulties, cold, clammy or mottled skin, drowsiness or loss of consciousness).

YOUR NOTES

....
....
....
....
....
....
....
....
....
....
....
....
....
....
....
....

YOUR NOTES

....
....
....
....
....
....
....
....
....
....
....
....
....
....
....
....

LOOKING AFTER YOURSELF

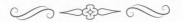

While you'll no doubt want
to throw everything into this
new exciting stage in your life,
try not to lose sight of your
own interests and well-being.
You may be a grandparent
now – but you're still you.

Grandmother–
grandchild relationships
are simple. Grandmas
are short on criticism
and long on love.

ANONYMOUS

GET PLENTY OF SLEEP

You're probably so thrilled by your gorgeous new grandchild that you'd spend every waking minute with them! But you'll be no use to them – or to anyone else – if you're exhausted. Try to stick to your usual routine rather than staying up late. If you're struggling to sleep because your mind's buzzing, try these useful ways to aid sleep:

◆ Limit your caffeine and sugar intake.

◆ Enjoy a relaxing evening bath with lavender essential oil drops in the water. Lavender helps relieve stress and is thought to promote sleep.

◆ Turn off all screens at least an hour before bedtime to help you switch off too.

◆ Allow 30 minutes to wind down before you get into bed.

A grandfather is someone with silver in his hair and gold in his heart.

ANONYMOUS

STAY ACTIVE

You may be a grandparent now, but that doesn't mean that you can stop taking care of yourself. You need plenty of energy to keep up with a little one, so stay active and healthy and you'll be able to enjoy yourself so much more. Try these ideas for low-impact exercise which you can fit in around visits to your grandchild.

◆ Go for a brisk walk – you could do this while pushing a pram!

◆ Head to your local pool to swim lengths or try aqua fit (water aerobics).

◆ Sign up for yoga – it's great for relieving stress as well as being a gentle workout.

Always check with your doctor first if you're embarking on a new fitness plan.

138

DON'T TAKE ON TOO MUCH

While you may love spending time with your grandchild and may want to help out as much as is humanly possible, it's important to know your limits.

If you're feeling stressed about being asked to do too much in the way of childcare, learn to say a polite but firm "no". It's okay to put yourself and your own health and well-being first. Be honest. Explain that it's all getting a bit too much and that, while you want to help, you can only do so much.

Come to a compromise. You may be happy to look after your grandchild at certain times – such as at weekends – but not in the evening. Do what's right for you.

DON'T FORGET THE LIFE YOU HAD BEFORE

You may be a grandparent now – but you're still you! It can be tempting to focus all your attention on that precious bundle, but it's important to carry on doing the things you did before baby arrived.

◆ If you're still working, make sure you're focused on your job when you're there.

◆ Don't stop calling your friends – and when you're with them, listen to their news too, even though it's tempting to bombard them with photos of your little darling.

◆ Don't abandon your hobbies. Whatever you enjoy doing in your spare time – whether it's painting, jogging, reading or something else – make time to carry on doing those things.

◆ If you're in a relationship, make time for your partner. Don't get so fixated on baby that you ignore everyone else.

RIDING THE ~ EMOTIONAL ~ ROLLER COASTER

It's not just the new parents who run a gamut of emotions. Grandparents can feel strung out too. Not only have you witnessed and supported the new parents through the highs and lows of pregnancy, you're now witnessing at close hand the first months of your grandchild's life. And those early days can be stressful!

There's so much to fret about, from growth charts to feeding issues and sleep patterns. But try to keep these fears in perspective. These worries are really for the parents to concern themselves with – if they need your help, you can be waiting with open arms.

You may also be feeling bowled over by just how much love you have for this little bundle, and be finding it hard to accept that you're the grandparent, not the parent. You might even ache for the days when you were a new parent yourself.

Be kind to yourself. Accept that time has moved on and things have changed. Allow yourself to take a step back when needed. Chat to a non-judgemental friend about how you feel. You'll probably discover that you're not the only new grandparent to have experienced this.

Finally, comfort yourself with the fact that being a grandparent means enjoying all the wonderful things about having a new baby in the family, while mainly avoiding the "not so fun" bits such as constant nappy changes and sleep deprivation!

Uncles and aunts, and cousins, are all very well, and fathers and mothers are not to be despised; but a grandmother, at holiday time, is worth them all.

Fanny Fern

What children need most are the essentials that grandparents provide in abundance. They give unconditional love, kindness, patience, humour, comfort, lessons in life. And, most importantly, cookies.

RUDOLPH GIULIANI

YOUR NOTES

....
....
....
....
....
....
....
....
....
....
....
....
....
....
....
....

YOUR NOTES

....
....
....
....
....
....
....
....
....
....
....
....
....
....
....

KEEPING IN TOUCH WHETHER YOU'RE NEAR OR FAR

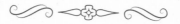

You may live on the other side of the world or just around the corner. Either way, it's important to nurture your relationship with your grandchild – and there are many ways to make this happen.

To show a child what has once delighted you, to find the child's delight added to your own, so that there is now a double delight seen in the glow of trust and affection, this is happiness.

J. B. PRIESTLEY

LONG-DISTANCE GRANDPARENTING – HOW TO COPE

It used to be common for entire families to live in the same area, and be in and out of each other's houses and each other's daily lives, but modern extended families today are often separated by miles.

If this is your situation, you may feel disappointed and sad. It's hard not being able to pop over for a quick cuddle or knowing that you won't be able to help with school runs in the future. But look for the positives. Advances in technology mean that it's easy to keep in touch with your grandchild. And while you might not be just around the corner, with the agreement of baby's parents, you can look forward to regular, longer visits to see your grandchild.

TECHNOLOGY – HOW
IT CAN HELP

It's useful to do your research so you know the best ways to keep in touch.

◆ Free live video calls – these can be streamed through Skype and WhatsApp. They're a great way for your family to connect – almost like being in the room together.

◆ Social media – Facebook and Instagram allow you to post photos and updates as well as seeing what your grandchild's parents have posted. Bear in mind that social media is never private so think before you post. As mentioned previously, always ask your grandchild's parents before posting photos of them online.

◆ Instant messaging – WhatsApp and Facebook Messenger allow you to send instant, free messages which can include digital photos, audio recordings and videos.

AVOIDING VISITS
BECOMING FRAUGHT

Whether you live near or far, it's useful to plan visits well in advance.

◆ Don't cram too much in – babies get overwhelmed very easily and don't need big days out. Simple days at home or short visits to a local park or café can be just as memorable.

◆ Go with the flow and expect the unexpected. Newborns don't follow a script and usually spend more time asleep than being entertaining!

◆ Respect your grandchild's routine. If baby goes to bed at 6 p.m. don't disrupt things.

◆ Don't overstay your welcome. If you've arranged to pop over for a couple of hours, resist the urge to hang around until dinner time. Exhausted new parents need their space!

◆ Offer to help. If you're staying for the afternoon or longer, be a useful visitor!

STRIKING A BALANCE
IF YOU'RE AROUND
THE CORNER

Living close to your grandchild is every doting grandparent's dream, right? But while regular contact nurtures a close and loving relationship, there are potential pitfalls too.

Make sure you establish boundaries early – check whether the new parents are happy for you to drop in unexpectedly or whether they would prefer some warning. Are they happy for you to turn up for meals and bath time or would they prefer you to be around just for playtime?

If you're over there a lot, make sure you're a useful visitor but don't fall into the trap of being roped into doing more childcare than you can manage.

I like to do nice things
for my grandchildren
– like buy them
those toys I've always
wanted to play with.

Gene Perret

AVOID SPOILING YOUR GRANDCHILD

You may consider it your right, as grandparent, to "spoil" your precious grandchild. You may argue that it isn't actually "spoiling" if you're simply lavishing them with love and attention. But if you're planning on showering them with gifts whenever you see them, it's wiser to exercise restraint.

Your role is that of a grandparent, not that of a magical Santa-like figure. For a start, it'll become very expensive! More importantly, your grandchild will associate you with material gifts rather than with love and kindness. Their parents are unlikely to thank you either, especially if you haven't checked with them first.

The handwriting
on the wall means
the grandchildren
found the crayons.

ANONYMOUS

YOUR NOTES

....
....
....
....
....
....
....
....
....
....
....
....
....
....
....
....

YOUR NOTES

THE TEN GOLDEN RULES OF GRANDPARENTING

1. Never announce the news before the new parents have had their moment!

2. Be supportive during the pregnancy.

3. Wait until you're invited to meet your new grandchild.

4. Offer a hand to hold during the overwhelming early days of parenthood.